Early Practice of Medicine by Women

Prof. Henry Carrington Bolton
Elizabeth and Emily Blackwell

Early Practice of Medicine by Women

LM Publishers

Part I

Early Practice of Medicine by Women[1]

In attempting to sketch the history of the entrance of women into the medical profession, we find the earlier periods obscured by a meagerness of material and a lack of sequence which our superficial researches have failed to supplement.

Isolated cases of gifted women attaining notable surgical skill and successfully pursuing the divine art of healing are recorded at various epochs in the history of the intellectual development of woman, but they occur at long intervals of time and in widely scattered chronicles. In the following pages we have not undertaken to present an exhaustive history or catalogue of female practitioners of medicine; we have simply collected a few scattered

---

[1] By Prof. Henry C. Bolton.

notices, and molded them into an outline to be hereafter filled up by a more competent hand.

These notices refer to the earlier history only, and by earlier history we mean the period prior to the establishment of medical schools for women, and to the present movement for their higher education. From the earliest times women have successfully grappled with a most difficult branch of medical science, gynecology, but long-existing and deep-seated prejudices prevented an extension of their practice, and save in exceptional cases they were forbidden both the acquirement of accurate and systematic knowledge and the exercise of their chosen vocation. So long as the practice of medicine formed a part of the priestly functions, as in ancient Egypt, the crafty guardians of superstition sedulously concealed their superior knowledge from an ignorant and credulous people, and especially from women. Yet the story of the birth of Moses shows that female gynecologists were not unknown to the Egyptians.

At a later period the Greeks thought to add dignity to the practice of medicine by forbidding it to slaves and (forsooth!) to women. During the middle ages, when every branch of science was more or less dishonored by degrading superstitions, we find women, as well as men, yielding to their influence and exercising the double calling of sorceress and healer of the sick; nor has the intelligence of the common people even in the nineteenth century reached such a height as to render the business of medical clairvoyant nugatory and profitless.

The invention of medicine was almost universally attributed by the ancients to the gods, and it is a curious fact that in both Egyptian and Grecian mythology we find female deities occupying important relations to the healing art. To the Egyptian deity Isis, the wife and sister of Osiris, peculiar medical skill was attributed, and a multitude of diseases were regarded as the effects of her anger. According to tradition she had given unequivocal proof of her power by the restoration of her son Orus to life. She was the reputed discoverer also of several remedies, and even as late as Galen the materia medica contained several compounds which bore her name: thus, in the symbolical language of the Egyptian priestly physicians, the vervain was called the "tears of Isis."

According to the annals of Grecian mythology, Hygeia, daughter of Æsculapius, the god of medicine, was worshiped in the temples of Argos as the goddess of health. In art, Hygeia is represented as a virgin wearing an expression of benevolence and kindness, and holding in one hand a serpent which is feeding from a cup in the other. She was regarded as the goddess both of physical and mental health, thereby personifying the aphorism, "Mens sana in corpore sano." The Greeks also ascribed medical power to Juno, who, under the name of Lucina, was held to preside over the birth of children, and to Ocyroe, daughter of the Centaur Cheiron, who was renowned for his skill in surgery and medicine. The sorceresses Medea and Circe were said to make use of herbs in their enchantments and for the purpose of counteracting the effects of poisons. These and similar fables probably preserve in allegoric form facts connected with the practice of medicine by women in the remotest antiquity. The writings of Homer have been examined to ascertain his testimony, but, with the exception of slight reference to woman's part in nursing wounded warriors, he contributes nothing to the subject under consideration.

The learned among the Celts, the Druids, were at the same time judges, legislators, priests, and physicians. By persuading the people that they maintained intimate relations with the gods, they succeeded in imposing their authority on the ignorant masses. "Their wives, who were called *Alraunes,* exercised the calling of sorceresses, causing considerable evil by their witchcraft, but caring for warriors wounded in battle. They gathered those plants to which they attributed magic virtues and they unraveled dreams" (Dunglison).

The first female practitioner who received a medical education appears to be Agnodice, a young Athenian woman who lived about 300 B. C. To satisfy her desire for knowledge she disguised herself in male attire, and, braving the fatal results of detection, dared to attend the schools of medicine forbidden to her sex. Among her instructors was numbered Herophilus, the greatest anatomist of antiquity and the first who dissected human subjects. After completing her studies, Agnodice preserved her disguise and practiced her chosen calling in the Grecian capital with great success, giving particular attention to the diseases of her own sex. The physicians of Athens becoming jealous of Agnodice's great reputation and lucrative practice, summoned her before the Areopagus, and accused her of abusing her trusts in dealing with female patients. To establish her innocence, Agnodice disclosed her sex, and her persecutors then accused her of violating the law prohibiting women and slaves from studying medicine, but the wives of the most influential Athenians arose in her defense and eventually obtained a revocation of the law.

The laws and customs of the Romans, as well as of the Greeks, were antagonistic to the entrance of women into the medical profession, yet Galen, Pliny, and others have preserved the names of a few distinguished in the art of healing: Phænarete, the mother of Socrates, Olympia of Thebes, Salpe, Sotira, Elephantis, Favilla, Aspasia, and Cleopatra. Of these, details are generally wanting. Scribonius Largus writes of an "honest matron" who cured several epileptic patients by an absurd remedy, and mentions having purchased of a woman a prescription for the cure of colic, the composition of which she had learned in Africa. Why Aspasia appears in this connection is not perfectly clear; the talented wife of Pericles, renowned as "a model of female loveliness," was doubtless too involved in affairs of state to undertake the absorbing cares of the medical profession. Cleopatra, the accomplished and luxurious Queen of Egypt, of whom so many marvels are related, is named among those women possessed of medical skill; she is reported to have compounded cosmetics and to have written on the art of preserving beauty, but this statement is probably no more worthy of credence than that of the infatuated alchemists of the middle ages, who would persuade us that Cleopatra was the fortunate possessor of the philosopher's stone and of the universal solvent. In proof of the former statement, they point to her personal attractions, unchanged by increasing years, and to her immense wealth; in proof of the latter, they rely with confidence on the well-known fable of the solution of the costly pearl at the extravagant banquet to Marc Antony.

In a Roman lady named Fabiola we find an early predecessor of Florence Nightingale. She was of the illustrious house of Fabius, and was celebrated in the fourth century for piety and charity. She is to be held in grateful remembrance as the founder of hospitals in Italy, and she is said to have personally nursed the sick at Ostia. The establishment of hospitals is commonly credited to the Emperor Julian, 362 A. D., with whom Fabiola was contemporary; perhaps she took an active part in the humane movement, and held a position analogous to that of lady manager in modern times.

Half a century later lived a woman justly distinguished for combining in one person a high degree of female loveliness, womanly virtue, and intellectual strength: though not occupied with the art of healing, we cannot pass in silence the accomplished Hypatia. Born at Alexandria in the latter part of the fourth century, the daughter of Theon, an eminent mathematician and philosopher, she soon excelled her father in these branches of learning. After profiting by profound studies under celebrated masters at Athens and Alexandria, she publicly taught philosophy at both these centers of culture. Gibbon writes of her, "In the bloom of beauty and in the maturity of wisdom, the modest maid refused her lovers and instructed her disciples." On Hypatia's inhuman murder at the instigation of the jealous Cyril and his fanatical followers, it is not here necessary to dwell.

The practice of medicine by women obtained to some extent during the middle ages. Under the influence of Mohammedan rule, women were placed in excessive isolation, and it is not surprising to find under these circumstances that certain women were skilled in attending to the requirements of their own sex. Thus Albucasis, of Cordova, one of the most skillful surgeons of the twelfth century, secured the services of properly instructed women for assistance in operations on females in which considerations of delicacy intervened. Avicenna also, writing of remedies for diseases of the eyes, mentions a collyrium compounded by a woman well versed in medical science. On the whole, however, the number of women instructed in medicine among the Arabs was very small, owing possibly to the inferiority to which women were condemned by Eastern usages.

In Christian countries the nuns as well as the priests attended to the healing of the sick as an act of charity and piety. Abelard, in the twelfth century, permitted the practice of surgery to those of the convent of the Paraclete, over which Héloïse presided. The most celebrated of the learned nuns was Hildegarde (A. D. 1098-1180), abbess of the convent of Rupertsberg, near Bingen on the Rhine. She compiled a sort of materia medica, which comprises a variety of superstitious remedies. Radegonde of France, the founder of a convent at Poitiers (died 587), the pious ascetic Elizabeth of Hungary (died 1231), Hedwigia, wife of Henry the Bearded, and other women who devoted themselves to the care of the sick, may be properly regarded as praiseworthy exemplars of Christian benevolence rather than educated practitioners of medicine.

In the famous school of medicine established at Salernura by Benedictine monks in the eleventh century, we find women taking an important part. Ordericus Vitalis, in his "Ecclesiastical History" (written about 1130), relates that an abbot eminent in natural sciences-, and especially distinguished in medicine, visited Salernum in the year 1059 for the purpose of discussing medical topics, and found no one erudite enough to reply to his propositions save a certain woman of great learning. This woman he does not name, but she is supposed to be the same as Trotula of Ruggiero, whose reputation at that period was world-wide. At Salernum, women were engaged in the preparation of drugs and cosmetics, and in the practice of medicine among persons of both sexes: such were Abella, author of two medical poems; Costanza Calenda, the talented and beautiful daughter of a skillful physician, under whose instructions she attained to a doctor's degree; Mercuriade, author of several treatises; Rebecca Guarna, Adelmota Maltraversa, and Marguerite of Naples, who obtained royal authority for practicing the medical art.

The ancient and honorable universities of Italy were, we believe, the first to recognize the capacity of women to give instruction of a high character. The University of Bologna, founded in 1116, was attended in the year 1250 by ten thousand students, engaged m the study of jurisprudence, of philosophy, and of medicine. "Here was first taught the anatomy of the human frame, the mysteries of galvanic electricity, and later the circulation of the blood." Here, too, were the earliest successful experiments in admitting women to occupy professorial chairs, for a long line of female professors taught in many departments of learning.

As early as the thirteenth century two women were numbered among the eminent professors of the University of Bologna, Accorsa Accorso and Bettisia Gozzadini, the former held the chair of Philosophy, the latter that of Jurisprudence. In the fourteenth century the lovely and learned Novella d'Andrea, daughter of a distinguished lawyer, often took her father's place in the professorial chair, and instructed his students in law. Of Novella it is reported that she was so beautiful that she lectured behind a curtain, "lest, if her charms were seen, the students should let their young eyes wander over her exquisite features and quite forget their jurisprudence." The rival University of Padua, founded in 1228, had also its female representatives. Of these the most distinguished was Elena Lucrezia Cornaro. This interesting woman was born at Venice, June 5, 1646, and at a very early age exhibited an extraordinary capacity for acquiring languages. She was familiar with French, Spanish, Latin, Greek, and Hebrew, besides her native Italian, and had some acquaintance with Arabic. While endowed by nature with poetical and musical talents, she possessed at the same time great perseverance and capacity for serious studies, and discoursed eloquently on abstruse topics in philosophy, mathematics, astronomy, and theology. At the age of thirty-two, the University of Padua conferred upon her the degree of Doctor of Philosophy. Cornaro seems never to have held any public position, being naturally of a retiring disposition, and moreover exceedingly devoted to the order of St. Benedict. After acquiring a European reputation, she died at the comparatively early age of thirty-eight (1684).

The beginning of the following century witnessed the birth of one of the most gifted women the world has ever seen. Laura Caterina Bassi was born at Bologna, October 31, 1711. She was the daughter of a distinguished lawyer and *littérateur,* and at a tender age manifested extraordinary precocity, being able while still a child to translate fluently most difficult Latin and Greek. Encouraged by her father, she pursued her studies under the guidance of eminent masters; she learned physiology and medicine with the erudite physician Gaetano Tacconi, mathematics with Manfredi, and natural philosophy with the disciples of Gassendi, and she astonished these profound philosophers by her talents. Laura Bassi studied for the pure love of knowledge, and had no ambition to seek public honors, but, to gratify the pardonable pride of a father as well as the earnest desires of her instructors, she consented to support a philosophical thesis before a learned audience of professors. This event took place on the 17th of April, 1732, before she had reached the age of twenty-one years. The occasion was made one of festivity by the whole city, who turned out to do her honor; the assemblage was presided over by two cardinals, Lambertini, afterward Pope Benedict XIV, and Grimaldi.

According to custom her thesis was opposed by seven learned men; to these she replied in elegant Latin with great success and amid the applause of the distinguished audience. A month later the degree of Doctor was conferred upon her, and she was honored by a position in the Faculty of Philosophy. The Senate subsequently bestowed upon her the chair of Physics, and commemorated the event by striking a medal which bore her own portrait. She held the professorship twenty-eight years with marked success, paying particular attention to mathematics and physics, also to *belles-lettres.* Several academies of learning elected her to membership. In 1738 she was married to J. J. Veratti, a physician, and became in the course of time the mother of twelve children. A learned French *littérateur* who visited Bologna in her day thus describes her appearance: "Laura Bassi has a countenance slightly marked with small-pox, but of a sweet and modest expression; her black eyes are sparkling, yet tranquil, and she is serious and composed in demeanor without affectation or vanity. Her memory is tenacious, her judgment sound, and her imagination active." She died in the year 1778, at the age of sixty-seven.

Laura Bassi does not seem to have pursued medical studies, and certainly never engaged in practice; but any account of the gifted women of Bologna who labored in this direction would be incomplete without a brief notice of Madame Veratti.

Contemporary with this interesting woman lived another, less gifted but scarcely less renowned. Anna Morandi was born at Bologna five years later than Laura Bassi, and died four years earlier. She became the wife of Giovanni Manzolini, a poor, hard-working maker of anatomical models. Manzolini was an expert painter and modeler in wax, and was employed by one Lelli to construct a series of anatomical models for the use of the professors in the Institute of Bologna. Anna not only aided her husband, but soon surpassed him in skill, and particularly in that scientific knowledge upon which the success of their joint labors so largely depended. About this time Giovanni Antonio Galli, a skillful surgeon and Professor of Gynecology, opened a school of obstetrics in his house, and, encouraged by him, Anna began to lecture on anatomy to private classes. In these lectures she not only imparted with peculiar talent the knowledge derived from her husband, but she also communicated many discoveries made by herself. So great was her skill in all dissections requiring delicacy of touch and minuteness of detail, and so clearly did she demonstrate both theoretically and practically the wonderful structure of the human body, that she rapidly acquired a European reputation, and her lecture-room was frequented by students of all countries.

In 1755 Anna Manzolini became a widow, and was left with very slender means of support, but her good qualities raised up friends who secured for her a comfortable subsistence. Though she received tempting offers from other Italian universities, and even from England and Russia, she preferred to remain in her native city, Bologna. Not long after her husband's death she was appointed to the chair of Anatomy in the Bologna Institute.

Anna Morandi-Manzolini enjoys the distinction of having been the first "to reproduce in wax such minute portions of the human body as the capillary vessels and the nerves." Her collection of anatomical models, still to be seen at the Institute of Science, bears silent testimony to her remarkable skill and accurate knowledge. "Her lectures were delivered in the fragrant cedar hall which is one of the modern sights of Bologna and in which Lelli's anatomical wooden figures supporting the canopy over the professorial chair attract general admiration." In the anatomical gallery of the university is to be seen her portrait in wax, modeled by herself at the request of many admiring friends. Anna Manzolini closed a laborious and honored life in 1774, at the age of fifty-eight years.

The city of Bologna, in the middle of the eighteenth century, saw three gifted women simultaneously occupying seats in the faculty of its ancient university. Besides Laura Bassi and Anna Morandi-Manzolini, of whom we have briefly spoken, Maria Gaetano Agnesi was equally distinguished.

Maria Agnesi was born at Milan, March 16, 1718. At an early age she manifested a remarkable facility for acquiring languages, and when only twenty years old was able to discourse in French, Spanish, German, Greek, and Hebrew, besides her mother-tongue. She displayed marked ability also in philosophy and mathematics, and while still young sustained one hundred and ninety-one theses which were afterward printed under the title "Propositiones Philosophicæ." In 1748 Agnesi published a treatise on algebra, including the differential and integral calculus, in which she displayed wonderful judgment and erudition. This work ("Instituzioni Analitichi") was afterward translated by Colson, the Lucasian Professor of Mathematics at Cambridge, and was used by the students of that university. In 1750 her father, who was Professor of Mathematics at the University of Bologna, fell sick, and she obtained permission of the good Pope Benedictus XIV to occupy her father's chair. In person Agnesi is said to have been beautiful, modest, and of pleasing manners. Her severe studies overtaxed her delicate frame, and shortly after she renounced the world and took refuge among the Blue Nuns at Bologna. In this nunnery she lived several years a devotee and an invalid; she died in 1799.

While Laura Bassi taught physics, Anna Morandi-Manzolini anatomy, and Maria Agnesi mathematics, in the Bolognese University, we might naturally expect the gentler sex to avail themselves of the opportunity of studying under their sisters' instructions. And such, in fact, was the case: the names of some of these students are recorded by the historian, many of whom received the degrees of Doctor of Philosophy and Doctor of Medicine. In 1799 Doctor Maria delle Donne appears as Professor of Medicine and Obstetrics; Clotilda Tambroni was Professor of the Greek Language and Literature, from 1793 to 1808. To these names should be added those of Novella Calderini, Maddalena Buonsignori, Dorotea Bocchi (who was both doctor and professor), Christina Roccati, Ph. D., Zaffira Ferretti, M. D., Maria Sega, M. D., and numerous graduates of Padua, Pavia, Ferrara, and other Italian universities.

Leaving the Italian Peninsula, which was so productive of remarkable personages, we will briefly examine the position of women practitioners of medicine in other parts of Europe.

Beaugrand states that the most ancient document extant relative to the organization of surgery in France forbids the practice of surgeons and of *female* surgeons who have failed to pass a satisfactory examination before the proper authorities. This paper bears the date 1311. References to female surgeons appear again in an edict of King John in 1352; from these documents it appears that women exercised the function of surgeon under legal authority. At a somewhat later period we find the calling of physician followed by women in Spain, Germany, and England.

In Spain, the Universities of Cordova, Salamanca, and Alcala honored many women with doctors' degrees. We note also the appearance at Madrid in 1587 of a learned medical work entitled "Nueva filosofia de la naturaleza del hombre," and published over the name Olivia del Sabuco. Of this person, however, nothing whatever is certainly known, and it has been conjectured that the name Olivia was a pseudonym assumed by some eminent physician.

In Germany many women cultivated medical science: Barbara Weintrauben was an author of no great merit; the Duchess Eleanor of Troppau, Catharina Tissheim, Helena Aldegunde, and Frau Erxleben are deserving passing notice. The last mentioned was one of the most successful female practitioners of the last century. Her maiden name was Dorothea Leporin, but she is best known as Frau Erxleben. Fräulein Leporin pursued her medical studies at the University of Halle, and obtained a diploma in 1734. She settled in the little town of Quedlinburg, at the foot of the Hartz Mountains, became the wife of the rector of the Church of St. Nicholas in the same place, industriously practiced her profession, and became eminent for her skill and learning. Her son, J. C. P. Erxleben, inherited from his mother a love of scientific pursuits and became a distinguished naturalist and professor in the University of Göttingen.

In England, Anna Wolley and Elizabeth of Kent were occupied with the preparation of drugs as early as the seventeenth century, and both published works on medical subjects.

In this hasty and superficial sketch of the history of the early practice of medicine by women we would not be true to the facts if we omitted mention of certain ignorant and vulgar women who assumed medical knowledge and medical skill to impose upon a too credulous public. That avaricious women, fond of notoriety and careless of their reputation, should imitate the methods adopted in every age by unprincipled men, is not surprising though it may be mortifying. To this class belonged Louise Bourgeois, nurse to Marie de' Medici, the Queen of Henry IV of France; though an ignorant charlatan, she acquired extraordinary influence over her royal patroness, and her career abounds in curious, eventful episodes. She was the author of several medical treatises on the diseases of women, one of which was published at Paris in 1617.

A century later another female practitioner flourished, of whom women have no reason to be proud. In the year 1738 Mrs. Joanna Stephens proclaimed in London that she had discovered a sovereign remedy for a painful disease. Notwithstanding her gross ignorance and vulgar demeanor, she secured a large circle of patients from among the upper and wealthy classes, and, after enriching herself by enormous fees drawn from their credulity, she proposed to make her medical discovery public in consideration of the modest sum of twenty-five thousand dollars. A subscription was started for this purpose and enthusiastically taken up; the clergy, lords, and ladies, with an inexplicable infatuation, hastened to add their names to the list of subscribers. Failing, however, to raise so large a sum of money, Mrs. Stephens's friends obtained a grant of the desired amount from Parliament. The certificate testifying to the "Utility, Efficacy, and Dissolving Power of the Medicines," bears the date March 5, 1739, and is signed by twenty justices. These dearly purchased remedies were three in number, "a Powder, a Decoction, and Pills." The powder consisted of calcined egg-shells and snails; the decoction was a disgusting mixture of herbs, soap, and honey, boiled in water; and the pills were made of "calcined wild-carrot seeds, burdock-seeds, ashen keys, hips, and haws—all burned to a blackness—soap and honey."

Contemporary with Mrs. Stephens lived another impostor, Mrs. Mapp, sometimes known as "Crazy Sally of Epsom," and described as an "enormously fat, ugly creature, accustomed to frequent country fairs, about which she loved to reel, screaming, abusive, and in a state of beastly intoxication." This attractive lady was by profession a bone-setter, and was patronized by patients of rank and wealth, who sought her charily bestowed favors with ill-disguised contempt of her person. The town authorities of Epsom greatly esteemed Mrs. Mapp, or, perhaps we should say, highly valued the benefit the town derived from the influx of wealthy patients, and they offered her the sum of five hundred dollars per annum if she would continue to reside in the town.

The first half of this century has witnessed the career of a few women eminent in the art of healing; in France Madame La Chapelle had an extensive gynecological practice, and Madame Boivin attained to such distinction that she was honored with the degree of Doctor of Medicine by the University of Marburg. In Germany Charlotte Heidenreich and Fran Heiland, her step-mother, were similarly honored with doctors' diplomas.

It is the glory of America that she is distinguished above all countries not only as the cradle of liberty but also as the foster-mother of the intellectual advancement of women. Yet this has not always been the case; in the early chronicles of the colonists (themselves refugees from persecution) we find, strangely enough, many laws of an exacting and repressive character, some of which were aimed directly at the ambition and zeal of women. In the famous Blue Laws of Connecticut the following curious entry occurs under the date of March, 1638: "Jane Hawkins, the wife of Richard Hawkins, had liberty till the beginning of the third month called May, and the magistrates (if shee did not depart before) to dispose of her; and in the mean time shee is not to meddle in surgery or phisick, drinks, plaisters or oyles, nor to question matters of religion except with the Elders for satisfaction." (*"True Blue Laws of Connecticut,"* by J. H. Trumbull, 1876.)

A hundred and forty years later we find marked progress in liberality in the State of Connecticut. As early as 1773, in the town of Torrington, Litchfield County, two women were greatly honored and much sought for on account of their remarkable skill as accoucheuses. The first of these, Mrs. Jacob Johnson, to quote the historian of Torrington (Rev. Samuel Orcutt), was as thoroughly known and trusted in her profession as any physician that was ever in the town. "She rode on horseback, keeping a horse for the special purpose, and traveling night and day, far and near," to meet her engagements. "She kept an account of the number of cases she had, and the success of the patients, and the new-comers, and of these last there is at least one living in the town. In the midst of her usefulness she was removed by death, and it became a great inquiry, 'Who will take the place of Granny Johnson?'" This question was answered in the person of Mrs. Huldah Beach, daughter of Aaron Loomis, Jr., more successfully than was anticipated. Mrs. Beach became as celebrated in her calling as Granny Johnson, and continued to attend to her professional duties until an advanced age. She was a woman of remarkably fine personal appearance and decided dignity of carriage, yet marked kindliness of manner. Her intellectual strength and ability were perceptible to everyone, and she in consequence commanded great respect in all classes of society, and won the confidence of the people so that but few calls were made on any other physician in her specialty, on the western side of the town. She also rode as far as Winchester, Goshen, and Litchfield.

Dr. Orcutt, whose "History of Torrington" has furnished us with these particulars, remarks in this connection, "Many have imagined that, in the practice of medicine by women, a new era has arrived, but in this there is only a 'restoration of the lost arts.'"

Our allotted task is completed, yet we cannot close this address without a brief survey of the present period, in which the facilities afforded women in all branches of learning contrast strongly with the formerly wellnigh insurmountable impediments and obstacles.

Women desirous of acquiring medical knowledge are no longer obliged to disguise themselves in male attire like Agnodice the Athenian, nor are practitioners liable to suffer the penalties of the law for their works of benevolence and charity. In 1880 the young woman with aspirations for intellectual culture finds open to her such excellent training-schools as Holyoke, Wells, and Rutgers, such-noble institutions as Vassar, Smith, and Wellesley. Does she not shrink from contact with her brothers, she may gain entrance into many universities, either expressly founded in a liberal spirit, as Oberlin, Cornell, and Ann Arbor, or which have yielded to the steady pressure of public opinion, and now open their doors more or less widely to the gentler sex. To enumerate the latter would be tedious and unprofitable; suffice it to say that even venerable and aristocratic Harvard has lately joined the number, and our own Columbia, should her President's views prevail, will not be slow to follow.

The young woman who seeks intellectual training of a more technical character, with a view to adopting a professional career, will find many avenues opening up with constantly increasing privileges and facilities. The student in art, thanks to the philanthropy of our venerable citizen, Peter Cooper, can, without incurring expense, acquire a knowledge of designing or of wood-engraving which will hardly fail to secure for her a competence. The student in biology will receive her share of attention at a summer school of science on our Atlantic seaboard, or held in connection with some enterprising institution of learning. The student in pharmacy and chemistry can conduct her researches on an equality with men, or, if she prefer, in laboratories controlled and officered in large part by women themselves.

The student in medicine now gains access to medical colleges in nearly every State in the Union, and the legitimacy of her pursuit as well as her ability to grapple with it gains increasing advocates. "She is no longer regarded as too good and too stupid to study medicine." The candidate for medical honors also finds in Boston, Philadelphia, New York, and Chicago, well-appointed schools of medicine especially adapted to her needs, with corps of trained and sympathizing instructors ready to lend a helping hand.

Looking across the Atlantic, we find countries so lately intolerant of the intellectual advancement of woman at last yielding, not always gracefully, to the inevitable. The little republic of Switzerland and the mighty empire of Russia have for many years manifested practical sympathy with the cause; and now, slowly yet surely, conservative England begins to recognize the fact that the Anglo-Saxon race, with its boasted love of liberty, has been neglectful of its duty to womankind.

To trace any more fully the history of the recent period does not fall within the province of our address; we look to the pioneers of this movement who are still with us for an exhaustive and authentic record such as participators and eye-witnesses alone can supply.

Part II : Testimony

Medicine as a Profession for Women[2]

In inviting consideration to the subject of medicine as an occupation for women, it is not a simple theory that we wish to present, but the results of practical experience. For fourteen years we have been students of medicine; for eight years we have been engaged in the practice of our profession in New York; and during the last five years have, in addition, been actively occupied in the support of a medical charity. We may therefore venture to speak with some certainty on this subject; and we are supported by the earnest sympathy of large numbers of intelligent women, both in England and America, in presenting this subject for the first time to the public.

---

[2] by Elizabeth Blackwell and Emily Blackwell.

The idea of the education of women in medicine is not now an entirely new one; for some years it has been discussed by the public, institutions have been founded professing to accomplish it, and many women are already engaged in some form of medical occupation. Yet the true position of women in medicine, the real need which lies at the bottom of this movement, and the means necessary to secure its practical usefulness and success, are little known. We believe it is now time to bring this subject forward and place it in its true light, as a matter not affecting a few individuals only, but of serious importance to the community at large; and demanding such support as will allow of the establishment of an institution for the thorough education of women in medicine.

When the idea of the practice of medicine by women is suggested the grounds on which we usually find sympathy expressed for it are two. The first is, that there are certain departments of medicine in which the aid of *women* physicians would be especially valuable to women. The second argument is, that women are much in need of a wider field of occupation, and if they could successfully practice any branches of medicine it would be another opening added to the few they already possess. In some shape or other, these two points are almost universally regarded (where the matter has been considered at all) as the great reasons to be urged in its behalf.

Now, we believe that both these reasons are valid, and that experience will fully confirm them; but we believe also that there is a much deeper view of the question than this; and that the thorough education of a class of women in medicine will exert an important influence upon the life and interests of women in general, an influence of a much more extended nature than is expressed in the above views. The question of the real value to the community of what women may do in medicine is an eminently practical matter, for upon it is based the aid which they may ask for its accomplishment; and upon the position of women in medicine depends the kind and extent of education which should be given to fit them for it. A great deal of well-meant effort has been, and is still being expended upon the institutions which have been established for this purpose. Sometimes we have heard much discouragement expressed at the slight result that has followed from them; while, on the other hand, it is often said, "after all, it is a matter for women to settle for themselves, if they can be doctors, and want to, they will find the way to do it, there is no need of doing anything in the matter." Now as I have said, we believe it to be by no means a matter concerning only the limited number of women who may be actually engaged in the pursuit itself; and it is also certain that to insure the success of the work it is not enough that women should wish to study, the cooperation and support of public sentiment is needed to enable them to do so. We hope, by showing the value of the work, to prove it to be the interest of the community to carry it out; and we desire to show the means by which this may be done.

Let me then say a few words on the influence which would be exerted on society by the opening of medicine as a profession to women. The interests and occupations of women, as they actually are at present, may be referred to four distinct forms of effort: Domestic life; the education of youth; social intercourse, and benevolent effort of various kinds. All these avocations, by unanimous consent, are especially under the superintendence of women, and every woman, as she takes her place in society, assumes the responsibility of participation in some of them.

While these pursuits have always formed the central interest of the majority of women, their character, and the requirements which they make for their proper performance, have widened, with the advance of modern society, in a remarkable degree. Social intercourse—a very limited thing in a half civilized country, becomes in our centres of civilization a great power, establishing customs more binding than laws, imposing habits and stamping opinions, a tribunal from whose judgment there is hardly an appeal. All who are familiar with European life, and the life of our great cities, know what an organized and powerful force it ever tends to become.

In like manner, benevolent efforts have little influence in new countries, but in Europe, especially in England, the extent of such work, and the amount of it which is done by women would be incredible, did we not see here, in our midst, the commencement of a similar state of things.

Domestic life is not less affected by the growth of the age; the position and duties of the mother of a family call for very different qualifications, in the wide and complicated relations of the present, from what was needed a century ago.

Now it is evident that the performance of all these forms of work, extended and organized as they are, is in its practical nature a business requiring distinct knowledge and previous preparation, as much as actual trades and professions. This fact would be more commonly recognized were it not that there is so much moral and spiritual life interwoven into woman's work by the relations upon which it is founded, and out of which it grows, as to make it more difficult to separate this business aspect of her work from her personal life, than is the case with the business life of men; consequently its practical character is too often considered entirely subordinate, or lost sight of. Every woman, however, who brings thought and conscience to the performance of everyday duties, soon realizes it in her own experience. The wider the view she takes of life, the higher her ideal of her domestic and social relations, the more keenly she will feel the need of knowledge with regard to this matter of fact basis upon which they rest. The first and most important point in which she will feel the want of this previous training will be in her ignorance of physiological and sanitary science, in their application to practical life; of the laws of health and physical and mental development; of the connection between moral and physical conditions, and the influences which our social and domestic life exert upon us. These and similar questions will meet her at every step, from the commencement of her maternal life, when the care of young children and of her own health bring to her a thousand subjects of perplexity, to the close of her career, when her children, assuming their positions as men and women, look to her as their natural counsellor.

It may be said, at first sight, that in these things it is not so much knowledge as common sense and earnestness that is wanted; that as health is the natural condition, it will be secured by simply using our judgment in not positively disregarding what our natural instincts teach us in regard to our lives. This would be true if civilization were a simple state directed by instinct; but every advance in social progress removes us more and more from the guidance of instinct, obliging us to depend upon reason for the assurance that our habits are really agreeable to the laws of health, and compelling us to guard against the sacrifice of our physical or moral nature while pursuing the ends of civilization.

From the fact, then, that our lives must be directed more by reason than instinct, arises at once the necessity for a science of health, and that comprehension of it which will lead to its daily application. Take in illustration the simplest physical need, that which is most completely instinctive in its character—the question of food. Animals make no mistake on this point, being governed infallibly by instinct, but what conflicting theories it has given rise to among men! It is very rare to find among women, the heads of families, any clear idea of what are the requisites for a healthy table; and what is true of this very simple material want is still more so with regard to higher questions of physical law, those more intimately connected with the intellect and affections, and the family and social relations growing out of them. Nothing is more striking in a wide observation of daily life than the utter insufficiency of simple common sense to secure wise action in these matters. Numbers of people, of very good common sense in other things, violate the fundamental laws of health without knowing it; and when they think upon the subject they are just as likely to follow some crude popular theory as to find out the truth.

That progress is needed in sanitary matters is widely admitted; sanitary conventions are held; the medical profession and the press are constantly calling attention to defects of public and private hygiene, pointing out the high rate of mortality amongst children, etc.; but it is far from being as generally recognized how essential to progress it is that women, who have the domestic life of the nation in their hands, should realize their responsibility, and possess the knowledge necessary to meet it.

In education, as in domestic life, the same necessity for hygienic knowledge exists. Statistics show that nine-tenths of our teachers are women, and it is obviously a matter of great importance that they should be familiar with the nature and needs of the great body of youth which is intrusted to their care. It is not possible that our systems of education should be really suited to childhood, training its faculties without cramping or unduly stimulating the nature, unless those by whom this work is done understand the principles of health and growth upon which school training should be based. Our school education ignores, in a thousand ways, the rules of healthy development; and the results, obtained with much labor and expense, are gained very generally at the cost of physical and mental health.

If, then, it be true that health has its science as well as disease; that there are conditions essential for securing it, and that every day life should be based upon its laws; if, moreover, women, by their social position, are important agents in this practical work, the question naturally arises, how is this knowledge to be widely diffused among them? At present there exists no method of supplying this need. Physiology and all branches of science bearing upon the physical life of man are pursued almost exclusively by physicians, and from these branches of learning they deduce more or less clear ideas with regard to the conditions of health in every-day life. But it is only the most enlightened physicians who do this work for themselves; a very large proportion of the profession, who are well acquainted with the bearing of this learning upon disease, would find it a difficult matter to show its relation to the prevention of disease, and the securing of health, by its application to daily life. If this be the case with regard to physicians, it must evidently be impossible to give to the majority of women the wide scientific training that would enable them from their own knowledge to deduce practical rules of guidance. This must be done by those whose avocations require wide scientific knowledge—by physicians. Yet the medical profession is at present too far removed from the life of women; they regard these subjects from such a different stand-point that they cannot supply the want. The application of scientific knowledge to women's necessities in actual life can only be done by women who possess at once the scientific learning of the physician, and as women a thorough acquaintance with women's requirements—that is, by women physicians.

That this connecting link between the science of the medical profession and the every-day life of women is needed, is proved by the fact that during the years that scientific knowledge has been accumulating in the hands of physicians, while it has revolutionized the science of medicine, it has had so little direct effect upon domestic life. Twenty years ago, as now, their opinion was strongly expressed with regard to the defects in the adaptation of modern life and education to the physical well being of society, and particularly of its injurious results to women. Yet, as far as these latter are concerned, no change has been effected. In all such points women are far more influenced by the opinions of society at large, and of their elder women friends, than by their physician, and this arises from the fact that physicians are too far removed from women's life; they can criticize but not guide it. On the other hand, it is curious to observe that, as within the last few years the attention of a considerable number of women has been turned to medicine, the first use they have made of it has been to establish a class of lecturers on physiology and hygiene for women. They are scattered all over the country; the lectures are generally as crude and unsatisfactory as the medical education out of which they have sprung; but the impulse is worthy of note, as showing the instinctive perception of women, as soon as they acquire even a slight acquaintance with these subjects, how directly they bear upon the interests of women, and the inclination which exists to attempt, at least, to apply them to their needs. As teachers, then, to diffuse among women the physiological and sanitary knowledge which they need, we find the first work for women physicians.

The next point of interest to be noticed is the connection of women with public charities and benevolent institutions.

In all civilized nations women have always taken an active share in these charities; indeed, if we include those employed in the subordinate duties of nurses, matrons, etc., the number of women actually engaged would much outnumber that of men. How large a part of the character of these institutions, and of the influence exerted by them upon society, is dependent upon this great body of women employed in them and connected with them, may readily be imagined. Yet it is certain, and admitted by all who have any acquaintance with the matter, that this influence at present is far from being a good one. It is well known how much the efficiency of women as managers or supporters of public institutions is impaired by the lack of knowledge and practical tact to second their zeal; and business men who have dealings with them in these relations are very apt to regard them as troublesome and uncertain allies, rather than as efficient coworkers. With those employed in the active care of the institutions the case is still worse; the very term hospital nurse conveys the idea of belonging to a degraded class.

How to obviate this great evil has become an important question. In England, where all public institutions, hospitals— civil and military—workhouses, houses for reformation, prisons, penitentiaries, etc., form a great system, dealing with the poorer classes to an immense extent, and having a social importance too serious to be overlooked, the question has assumed sufficient weight to be discussed earnestly by government and the public at large.

In Catholic countries this is accomplished to a certain extent—that is, as far as the domestic and nursing departments are concerned—by the religious orders, the sisters of charity and others. Everyone who is familiar with such institutions must have been struck by the contrast between the continental and English hospitals, etc., caused by this one thing, by the cheerful and respectable home-like air of well-managed French establishments, as compared with the gloomy, common aspect of even wealthy English or American charities; and must have observed the salutary influence upon patients, students, and all connected with these places, of the presence and constant superintendence of women who, instead of being entirely common and subordinate, are universally regarded with respect and confidence, and by the poorer classes almost with veneration.

It is very common among both Catholics and Protestants to consider these sisterhoods as the result entirely of religious enthusiasm, and to assert that large bodies of women can only be induced to accept these occupations, and carry them out in this efficient manner from this motive. When efforts have been made in England and Germany to establish anything of the kind among Protestants, it is always to the religious element that the appeal has been made. Many such efforts have been made, with more or less success, in Germany. In England, the results have been very imperfect, and have entirely failed to secure anything approaching in practical efficiency to the Catholic sisterhoods.

Now these failures are very easily comprehended by anyone who has seen much of these sisters in actual work, for such persons will soon perceive that the practical success of these orders does not depend upon religious enthusiasm, but upon an excellent business organization. Religious feeling there is among them, and it is an important aid in filling their ranks and keeping up their interest; but the real secret of their success is in the excellent opening afforded by them for all classes of women to a useful and respected social life. The inferior sisters are plain, decent women, nothing more, to whom the opportunity of earning a support, the companionship, protection and interest afforded by being members of a respected order, and the prospect of a certain provision for age, are the more powerful ties to the work, from the fact that they are generally without means, or very near connexions, and would find it difficult to obtain a better or so good a living. The superior sisters are usually women of character and education, who, from want of family ties, misfortune, or need of occupation, find themselves lonely or unhappy in ordinary life; and to them the church, with its usual sagacity in availing itself of all talents, opens the attractive prospect of active occupation, personal standing and authority, social respect, and the companionship of intelligent co-workers, both men and women—the feeling of belonging to the world, in fact, instead of a crippled and isolated life. For though it is common to speak of the sisters as renouncing the world, the fact is, that the members of these sisterhoods have a far more active participation in the interests of life than most of them had before. No one can fully realize the effect this has upon them, unless they have at once seen them at their work, and are aware how welcome to great numbers of women would be an active, useful life, free from pecuniary cares, offering sympathy and companionship in work and social standing to all its members, with scope for all talents, from the poorest drudge to the intelligent and educated woman—an offer so welcome as to be quite sufficient to overcome the want of attraction in the work itself at first sight.

As we have said, every effort so far to introduce a corresponding class of women into English institutions has proved a failure, for there is no such organization in external life in Protestant churches as there is in the Catholic; it is contrary to the genius of the nation; and the same results would certainly follow in America.

The only way to meet the difficulty, to give a centre to women who are interested in such efforts, and to connect intelligent women with these institutions, is to introduce women into them as physicians. If all public charities were open to well educated women physicians, they would exert upon them the same valuable influence that is secured by the presence and services of the superiors of these orders; they would bring in a more respectable class of nurses and train them, which no men can do; they would supervise the domestic arrangements, and give the higher tone of womanly influence so greatly needed.

They would be at the same time a connecting link between these establishments and women in general life, enlisting their interest and active services in their behalf, far more effectually than could be done by any other means. A real and great want would thus be supplied, and one which no other plan yet proposed has proved at all adequate to meet.

We come now to the position of women in medicine itself. The fact that more than half of ordinary medical practice lies among women and children, would seem to be, at first sight proof enough that there must be here a great deal that women could do for themselves, and that it is not a natural arrangement that in what so especially concerns themselves, they should have recourse entirely to men. Accordingly we find that, from the very earliest ages, a large class of women has always existed occupying certain departments of medical practice. Until within half a century, a recognized position was accorded to them, and midwives were as distinct a class, as doctors. Even now, in most European countries, there are government schools for their instruction, where they are most carefully trained in their own speciality. This training is always given in connexion with a hospital, of which the pupils perform the actual practice, and physicians of standing are employed as their instructors. In Paris, the great hospital of La Maternité, in which several thousand women are received annually, is entirely given up to them, and Dubois, Professor of Midwifery in the medical school of Paris, is at the head of their teachers. Until within a few years, it was common for eminent French physicians to receive intelligent midwives as their private pupils, and take much pains with their education. They were also admitted to courses of anatomical instruction in the *Ecole Pratique*, and an immense amount of practice was in the hands of these women. The whole idea of their education, however, planned and molded entirely by men, was not to enable these women to do all they could in medicine, but to make them a sort of supplement to the profession, taking off a great deal of laborious poor practice, and supplying a certain convenience in some branches where it was advantageous to have the assistance of skilful women's hands. With the advance of medical science, however, and its application to all these departments of medicine, this division of the directing head, and the subordinate hand, became impossible. Physicians dismissed, as far as possible, these half-educated assistants, excluded them from many opportunities of instruction under their authority, and in the government schools, which popular custom still upholds, they have materially curtailed their education. Nor is it possible or desirable to sanction the practice of any such intermediate class. The alternative is unavoidable of banishing women from medicine altogether, or giving them the education and standing of the physician. The broad field of general medical science underlies all specialities, and an acquaintance with it is indispensable for the successful pursuit of every department. If the popular instinct that called women so widely to this sort of work represent a real need, it can only be met now by a class of women whose education shall correspond to the wider requirements of our present medical science.

Moreover, experience very soon shows that it is not these special branches of practice that will chiefly call for the attention of women in medicine. The same reason which especially qualifies women to be the teachers of women, in sanitary and physiological knowledge, viz., that they can better apply it to the needs of women's life, holds good in regard to their action as physicians. So much of medical practice grows out of everyday conditions and interests, that women who are thoroughly conversant with women's lives will, if they have the character and knowledge requisite for the position, be as much better qualified in many cases to counsel women, as men would be in similar circumstances to counsel men. At present, when women need medical aid or advice, they have at once to go out of their own world, as it were; the whole atmosphere of professional life is so entirely foreign to that in which they live that there is a gap between them and the physician whom they consult, which can only be filled up by making the profession no longer an exclusively masculine one. Medicine is so broad a field, so closely interwoven with general interests, dealing as it does with all ages, sexes, and classes, and yet of so personal a character in its individual applications, that it must be regarded as one of those great departments of work in which the cooperation of men and women is needed to fulfill all its requirements. It is not only by what women will do themselves in medicine, but also by the influence which they will exert on the profession, that they will lead it to supply the needs of women as it cannot otherwise.

Our own experience has fully proved to us the correctness of this view. We find the practice, both public and private, which comes naturally to us is by no means confined to any special departments, and where patients have sufficient confidence in us to consult us for one thing, they are very apt to apply in all cases where medical aid is needed. The details of our medical work during the number of years that we have been connected with the profession cannot be given to the public, but they have fully satisfied us that there will be the same variety in the practice of women as exists in that of men; that individual character and qualification will determine the position in practice, rather than pre-conceived ideas with regard to the position; and that there is no department in which women physicians may not render valuable services to women.

It is often objected to this idea of professional and scientific pursuits for women that it is too much out of keeping with their general life, that it would not harmonize with their necessary avocations in domestic and social life; that the advantages to be gained from the services of women physicians would not compensate for the injurious effect it would have upon the women themselves who pursued the profession, or the tendency it might have to induce others to undervalue the importance of duties already belonging to them.

This objection, the prominent one which we usually meet, appears to us based on an entire misapprehension of what is the great want of women at the present day. All who know the world must acknowledge how far the influence of women in the home, and in society, is from what it should be. How often homes, which should be the source of moral and physical health and truth, are centers of selfishness or frivolity! How often we find women, well meaning, of good intelligence and moral power, nevertheless utterly unable to influence their homes aright. The children, after the first few years of life, pass beyond the influence of the mother. The sons have an entire life of which she knows nothing, or has only uneasy misgivings that they are not growing up with the moral truthfulness that she desires. She has not the width of view—that broad knowledge of life, which would enable her to comprehend the growth and needs of a nature and position so different from hers; and if she retain their personal affection, she cannot acquire that trustful confidence which would enable her to be the guardian friend of their early manhood. Her daughters also lack that guidance which would come from broader views of life, for she cannot give them a higher perception of life than she possesses herself. How is it, also, with the personal and moral goodness attributed to woman, that the tone of social intercourse, in which she takes so active a part, is so low? That, instead of being a counterpoise to the narrowing or self-seeking spirit of business life, it only adds an element of frivolity and dissipation.

The secret of this falling short from their true position is not a want of good instinct, or desire for what is right and high, but a narrowness of view, which prevents them from seeing the wide bearing of their duties, the extent of their responsibilities, and the want of the practical knowledge which would enable them to carry out a more enlightened conception of them. The more connections that are established between the life of women and the broad interests and active progress of the age, the more fully will they realize this wider view of their work. The profession of medicine which, in its practical details, and in the character of its scientific basis, has such intimate relations with these every-day duties of women, is peculiarly adapted as such a means of connection. For what is done or learned by one class of women becomes, by virtue of their common womanhood, the property of all women. It tells upon their thought and action, and modifies their relations to other spheres of life, in a way that the accomplishment of the same work by men would not do. Those women who pursued this life of scientific study and practical activity, so different from woman's domestic and social life and yet so closely connected with it, could not fail to regard these avocations from a fresh stand-point, and to see in a new light the noble possibilities which the position of woman opens to her; and though they may be few in number, they will be enough to form a new element, another channel by which women in general may draw in and apply to their own needs the active life of the age.

We have now briefly considered the most important grounds on which the opening of the profession of medicine to women is an object of value to society in general, and consequently having a claim upon the public for aid in its accomplishment. Let me now state briefly what are the means needed for this purpose.

The first requirement for a good medical education is, that it be practical, i.e., that the actual care of the sick and observation by the bedside should be its foundation. For this reason, it must be given in connection with a hospital. This essential condition is equally required for the more limited training of the nurse, which, though perfectly distinct in character and object from that of the physician, agrees with it in this one point of its practical nature. In Europe, the shortest period of study required for a physician's degree is four years, and at least ten months of each year must be spent in attendance upon the course of instruction. This course comprises not only lectures on the different branches of medicine, but thorough practical study of chemistry, botany, anatomy, etc., in the laboratory, gardens, museums, etc. Attendance on the hospitals is also required, where, for several years, the student is occupied with subordinate medical and surgical duty. This hospital training is the foundation of their education, and the lectures are illustrative of it, not a substitute for it. In England, no medical school can confer a degree that has not attached to it a hospital of as many as one hundred beds. And in many of the best schools, as that of St. Bartholomew's, of London, the college department will only number forty or fifty students, who perform all the assistants' duty of a hospital of five hundred beds, with an out practice of eighty thousand patients annually. In America, though so extensive and thorough an education is not legally required, yet all students who attain any standing in the profession pass through essentially the same course, because nothing short of it will enable them to meet the responsibilities of practice with success.

The chief difficulty in the way of women students at present is, as it always has been, the impossibility of obtaining practical instruction. There is not in America a single hospital or dispensary to which women can gain admittance, except the limited opportunities that have been obtained in connection with the New York Infirmary. This difficulty met us during our own studies, and we were obliged to spend several years in Europe to obtain the facilities we needed. Even there, no provision is made for the admission of women, but there are so many great hospitals in both London and Paris that only those distinctly connected with medical schools are crowded with students. There are many large institutions attended by distinguished physicians, comparatively little frequented by them, and in these a lady, with good introductions, can, if she will give the time and patience, find good opportunities for study.

This troublesome and expensive method is still the only way in which a woman can obtain anything that deserves to be called a medical education, but it is evidently beyond the means of the majority of women. The instruction that they have hitherto been able to obtain in the few medical schools that have received them has been purely theoretical. It consists simply of courses of lectures, the students being rigorously excluded from the hospitals of the city, which are only open to men. Some three hundred women have attended lectures in these schools, the majority of them being intelligent young women, who would probably have been teachers had they not chosen this profession. They enter the schools with very little knowledge of the amount and kind of preparation necessary, supposing that by spending two or three winters in the prescribed studies they will be qualified to begin practice, and that by gaining experience in practice itself they will gradually work their way to success. It is not until they leave college, and attempt, alone and unaided, the work of practice that they realize how utterly insufficient their education is to enable them to acquire and support the standing of a physician. Most of them, discouraged, having spent all their money, abandon the profession; a few gain a little practical knowledge and struggle into a second-rate position. No judgment can be formed of women as physicians under such circumstances. It would be evidently an injustice to measure their capacity for such occupation by their actual success, when all avenues to the necessary instruction are resolutely closed to them.

Realizing the necessity of basing any system of instruction for women on actual practice, we resolved, seven years ago, to lay the foundation of such an institution as was needed. A number of well-known citizens expressed their approval of the undertaking, and kindly consented to act as trustees. We then took out a charter for a practical school of medicine for women. This plan was founded upon those of European hospital schools. It is as follows: To a hospital, of not less than one hundred beds, lectureships are to be attached, for the different branches of medical science, with clinical teachers to give instruction in the wards. The students should be connected with it for four years, and should serve as assistants in the house, and in out-door practice. Amongst the professorships attached to the hospital should be one of sanitary science, of which the object is to give instruction on the laws of health, and all points of public and private hygiene, so far as science and practical life have taught us with regard to them. This professor should also supervise the sanitary arrangements of the hospital itself, and should be the chief of the system of instruction for nurses. We believe that this professorship would be of real and important value, not only in giving the students a thorough acquaintance with the laws and conditions of health, and fully imbuing them with the idea that it is as much the province of the physician to aid in preventing as in curing disease, but also as affording to teachers and mothers the opportunity of obtaining that sort of knowledge which we have shown they so much need, and yet have no means of acquiring. In this hospital we would also establish a system of instruction for nurses. The plans for this instruction are based upon those drawn up by Miss Nightingale for her proposed nursing school in London,—plans, the result of her long and wide experience, which, unfortunately, her ill health will probably prevent her carrying out, but with which, though never yet published, we are well acquainted.

This is a slight sketch of the mode in which we wish to carry out the three-fold object of the institution, viz., the education of physicians, the training of nurses, and the diffusion of sanitary knowledge amongst women.

It is evident that to organize such a hospital school would be a costly undertaking. It could not be self-supporting, for students are generally barely able to pay for their own direct instruction; and the hospital foundation, the apparatus for teaching, and in the professorships, must be at least in part supported by endowment. It would require, therefore, a very large sum to organize such an institution of the size I have described, and it could not be efficiently carried out on a smaller scale, but could we awaken in the public a conviction of the value of the object, we believe that any amount really needed to accomplish it would be raised.

When we took out our charter we knew that, having few friends to aid in the effort, we must work gradually toward so large an end. We accordingly began the New York Infirmary, as a small dispensary, in a single room, in a poor quarter of the city, open but a few hours during the week, and supported by the contributions of a few friends. Three years ago we had grown sufficiently to take the house now occupied by the institution, N° 64 Bleecker street, and with the same board of trustees and consulting physicians we organized a small house department. This year the number of patients treated by the Infirmary is about three thousand seven hundred. Although the institution is much too small to enable us to organize anything like a complete system of instruction for students or nurses, we have received into the house some of the elder students from the female medical schools, and a few women who have applied for instruction in nursing. We have thus become more familiar with their needs, and better able to shape the institution toward meeting them.

Although we cannot yet realize the ultimate objects toward which we are working, the institution, even of its present size, is of very great value. In the first place, the fact that the entire medical practice of such an institution is performed by women is the best possible proof to the public of the possibility of the practice of women, since, being public in its character, its results are known, as those of private practice cannot be. Secondly, it is already a valuable medical centre for women. The practice of a public institution, however small, establishes connexions between those who conduct it and others engaged in various public charities; and from the relations thus formed we have already been able to obtain facilities for students in the city dispensaries, and in private classes, that could not be obtained had we not such a centre to work from. Indeed, so effectual has it proved already in this manner, that were it established on a permanent basis, we could, by its assistance, and our connexions with the profession here and in Europe, enable individual students, possessing the requisite means, to obtain a good medical education before the institution itself can offer the complete education which I have described.

It is, moreover, a charity which is of much value to poor women, as being the only one where they can obtain the aid of women physicians. We have only been able to keep a very small number of beds, but they are constantly occupied by a succession of patients, and we could fill a much larger number if we were able to support them. Our dispensary practice is constantly increasing.

We believe, therefore, that, quite independent of the broader work that may be ultimately accomplished, in its present shape as a charity to poor women, as a proof of women's ability to practice medicine, and as a medical centre for women, this institution is well worthy of support.

What we ask from those who are interested in the objects we have stated is to assist in raising a fund for endowment which shall place the institution on a secure foundation. It has hitherto been supported almost exclusively by the subscriptions of a few friends, who pledged themselves for certain sums during three years. It has been a principle of management distinctly laid down, that the infirmary should not go into debt or on credit; that every year's expenses should be collected in advance, and should never be allowed to exceed the sum in the treasury at its commencement. This rule will be steadily adhered to, and no extension of operations undertaken until the funds are actually collected for that purpose. But so long as we are obliged to collect the income by subscription only from year to year we are not able even to lease a house, or make any arrangement for more than one year, but are obliged to devote to the work of its material support the time and attention that should be given towards organizing and furthering the objects of the institution. New York is the true centre of medical education. One hundred and fifty thousand patients received free medical aid last year; no other city in the Union compares with this in its need of medical charity. It is here, therefore, that a college hospital for women should be established. We have been urged to commence this work in England, and offers of valuable aid have been made for this purpose. But this medical work has originated here, and we believe that it is better suited to the spirit of this than of any other country. As America, therefore, has taken the initiative in this medical reform, let us do the work well.

I said to English friends before I left them, "You must send us over students, and we will educate them in America to do the same work in England." The cordial reply was, "We will send them over if we cannot prevail upon you to return to us."

Now, therefore, America must help us to redeem the pledge of education which we have given in her behalf.

Help us to build up a noble institution for women, such an institution as no country has ever yet been blessed with, a national college hospital, in which all parts of the Union shall join. Let it not be a name merely, but a substantial fact, wisely planned and liberally endowed.

Surely this awakening desire of women to do their duty in the world more earnestly, and to overcome, for a great and good end, the immense difficulties which stand in their way, will enlist the sympathy and support of every generous man and woman.